COUCH POTATO FITNESS

COUCH POTATO FITNESS

HOW TO RUN YOURSELF FIT IN LESS THAN 10 MINUTES A DAY

Christina Schnohr, PhD

Dedication

I dedicate this book to my three children, Sofus, Juliane and Frederik, who keeps reminding me of why I want to stay in good shape.

Can I Help You?

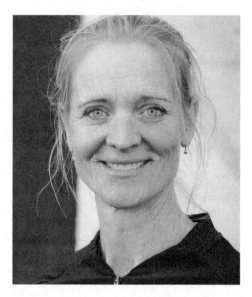

If you feel dedicated for training 1:1 time with me, I invite you to a ½ hour call to see if what I offer is what you are looking for

You can access my calendar below.

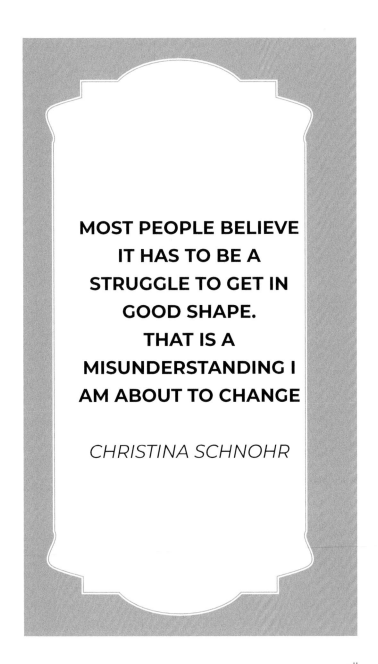

MOST PEOPLE BELIEVE
IT HAS TO BE A
STRUGGLE TO GET IN
GOOD SHAPE.
THAT IS A
MISUNDERSTANDING I
AM ABOUT TO CHANGE

CHRISTINA SCHNOHR

Contents

Come closer—and I'll let you in on a few secrets 1

    Why this book? 5

Open with a commitment
    (before you read any further) 11

    Stick to 1K a day – and no more 12

    Keep it simple! 15

    From now on you are an ATHLETE 20

Understanding The Psychology In Training 23

Claim Your New Love: Your Body 33

How You Overcome All The Excuses 37

    Do not let the excuses stop you 37

Persistence is power 47

Onekayaday 49

    Couch Potato Fitness is 1K a day 49

    Couch Potato Fitness in details 53

The Scientific Evidence 67

    Scientific evidence can motivate even more 67

All you need! 75

    The essential part of getting the work done! 75

The Healthy Lifestyle 79

Onward Journey 91

    Couch Potato Fitness (Online) Movement 92

Come closer—and I'll let you in on a few secrets

You are holding a book in your hands that is the product of a personal journey. I developed this training program for myself, after a rare crisis with my physical and mental well-being. After having spent a year developing it, and a year following it myself, I found out how well it worked – and how easy it was to share with others. People around me also experienced even better results than I had, mainly because the program was so simple. If it takes a lot of knowledge to explain something simple, I guess I am the right person to teach others about a simple running program. The program is so simple, that other personal trainers are skeptical. Most of the trainers hearing about it, do not believe that it can make such big changes, as it does. Which makes it even more fun to have created it! Before I describe the program to you, I would like you to get to know me a little, and to tell you a bit more about my background for making it.

What is important about me
This book is a product of my personal and long return to a strong and healthy body, after I gave birth in 2017. The

pregnancy and maternity leave with my third child had consumed more energy than I had, both because of sleep deprivation and because of the physical "adjustments", but I also experienced several relational problems with my close ones. In 2018, I felt completely drained and chronically low on battery.

I can see now that I was a physical and mental wreck.

I had also completely lost the drive for training, which was very new to me. For as long as I can remember, I have always enjoyed the feeling of a strong and healthy body. Wearing running shoes has been a dear memory to me since the age of 5, when I was put on the back of my mother's bike, and I joined the Running Club of the Copenhagen Heart Association. Their weekly training was where I had my running debut, and I remember how I ran as far as my legs would carry me – and used my seat on mother's bike as a resting place.

My family history with running goes back to before I was born. My father took the initiative to the oldest public run in Europe, The Eremitage

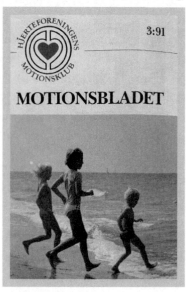

Photo: Peter Schnohr

Run in 1969, and that run has been a part of my family heritage – as well as a tradition to all the runners, who have been part of this run ever since 1969.

I started doing athletics when I was 12, and I beat national records from the very beginning.

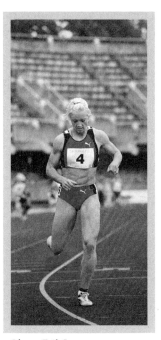

As a 16-year-old, I became the youngest Danish champion on the 100 and 200 meters at the national championships. When I stopped my career as a track and field athlete in 2001, I had won more national championships than any other Danish athlete. I gave birth to my first two children in 2004 and 2007, and after that, I suddenly enjoyed running longer distances,

Photo: Erik Laursen

as part of keeping healthy and happy. I ran my first marathon in 2010, in 2014, I ran my first ultramarathon, and in 2015, I ran a 100K race in England.

However, in 2018 something unexpected happened, and I suddenly found myself somewhere I had never been before.

I just did not feel like training. Or running! I was like a battery that needed charging. After I had worn out an unknown number of running shoes over the years, my shoes from ½ year ago were still new in my closet. I found myself with a complete lack of need to run.

I used all the practical tools and the academic knowledge I have gained over the years to find a way back to physical and mental surplus.

Admittedly, I had to dig deep, but the journey was worthwhile, because I found the simple principles, you will learn about in this book.

In 2020, I put the program into a system that I shared with some of my (male) friends, who had asked for my help. My first guinea pigs were busy CEOs in their forties, who were fed up with their poor physical condition and low energy levels. They called themselves couch potatoes, which inspired the name.

The feedback I got from everyone who even tried the training was overwhelmingly positive.

The results of theirs and several others' journeys, are described in the book, you hold in your hand.

My academic background is a PhD in health sciences, and I have been faculty at the University of Copenhagen, teaching epidemiology and disease prevention since 2005. My main interest is in health behavior and lifestyle changes. And I have a weak spot for the ones that are most inactive, as the health benefits are by far largest when this group becomes physically active. Additionally, the male gender is associated to shorter life spans, which have always urged me to support men to a healthier lifestyle.

I just LOVE to share my program with as many as possible, and I have transformed my knowledge and experience for it to benefit many people – including their families and colleagues.

Why this book?

I have never approved of inequality. And for as long I can remember, I have been cheering for the loosing team. During my years at university, we learned a lot about the shorter life span among men, and I have been curious about this ever since.

According to Statistics Denmark, Danish men can expect to live for approximately 80 years, while women can expect to become 84 years old. In Latvia, the difference is as much as 11 years between men and women!

It seems to be a universal challenge within public health to support men to become more active, and since there are no appropriate training programs to fit the lives of the hardworking family men, juggling several jobs both professionally and private, I am happy to deliver the perfect training program for him too – and many other busy or lazy people.

Couch Potato Fitness applies to everyone who wishes to become more physically active, and who does not know how to approach that task. It is of great advantage to already own a pair of running shoes.

In the chapter "The Scientific Evidence" you can read more about the causes of the difference between men and women's health, and here you can also read about what can be done.

Men smoke more, drink more, and are more overweight. They are also less likely to seek medical help when they get symptoms. Men are more often risk-takers, and they are more likely to die in accidents. But poor physical fitness is also contributing to shorter lives and poorer quality of life, and this is where I want to contribute.

I am hoping for better health among men, since improved fitness levels will both change the shorter life span, and change the many negative consequences associated to a life being overweight and living an unhealthy lifestyle. This book includes descriptions from men (and women), who – prior to following the program you are about to learn – had low self-esteem, were experiencing erectile dysfunction and were low on endurance, as part of being in a bad shape. I have also included descriptions from women, to serve as inspiration, as Couch Potato Fitness most certainly is not strictly for men.

Except the time around 2018 I have always trained in one form or another. In addition, I have always been wondering what the problem was with many people around me; training was something people talked a lot about but did not have time to get done. It is as if most people are carrying with them a constant bad conscience about not getting enough training done.

My basic drive to get my training done has always kept me in great shape for most of my life, which in my adult life has contrasted with many of my social relations. But as you have read about me already, I suddenly felt how a body without energy, pressure from my surroundings, and a pregnancy knocked me out to such an extent, that not even I felt like keeping in shape. This was when I understood what other people were talking about!

Now I understood why some people, day after day, would postpone their training, and how increasingly poorer physical fitness levels, would turn it into a vicious circle, to get back in shape.

I knew that there was a way out, and I kept looking for the solution. During my search, I was grateful for all I know about training, and after 1½ years of searching and trying out different solutions, I found the way that would get me back on track: Couch Potato Fitness.

You are holding the result in your hands

The training program is so simple, that you – just like everyone I have been coaching so far has expressed – may doubt that it will make a difference. But you will notice that it will!

Couch Potato Fitness is simple, but not easy. This book is my specific response to my view that training is over-thought, over-planned, and over-exercised. The book describes in detail, how little it takes for YOU to increase your physical fitness levels consistently.

If you follow the program and get through the three levels, the program consists of, you can expect big and remarkable changes, and an increased physical and mental fitness level. The first changes will occur already during the first days in the program.

32-year-old Karl could not recognize himself after the 15 weeks we worked together. When we started, he would never have imagined being able to run a 5K "with my wobbly body and bad knees". After he had completed Couch Potato Fitness he wrote to me a whole list of things, he would thank the program for. Of course, you must hear them:

Improved cardiovascular condition, higher self-worth, stronger physically, too large clothes, normalized blood pressure (after it had been slightly high), reduced alcohol intake ("in a good way"), more quality time with his children (because they joined him while he was running), and his wife had been inspired to also start following the program.

Just like many others I have been working with, Karl told me about the many excuses, he came up with to avoid training, and he pondered about that after the 15 weeks program.

The excuses were almost gone as the program evolved and training became part of his everyday life.

We are taking care of all the bad excuses in the chapter "How You Overcome All The Excuses".

Before we dig into the specifics of Couch Potato Fitness, I will explain a bit more background – as the training I would invite you to do is more a habit changing challenge, than an actual training program. But this is what works better in the long run. So you first need to know the crucial content of the next few chapters; the commitment that is needed, and the psychology behind it all.

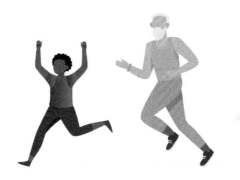

Open with a commitment (before you read any further)

You are reading these lines because you have decided to learn more about training. And I trust it is no coincidence, that you read these lines at exactly THIS point in time. You have your own reasons to have looked for a program that can support you to get started – or change your behavior.

I can assure you that you have come to the right place.

CONGRATULATIONS!

If you are waiting for a reason to start your training, you need to know that there is not going to be a reason. Do not think that you will wake up one morning thinking, "from today on, I am going to be someone who is training". This will not happen before you have been training for a while.

The feeling of wanting to train will come as soon as you have been doing it for a while, as you have then felt the benefits of what you are doing. Ironically, to the human species it is unnatural to be physically active unless we are in danger. The choice of making yourself out of breath and sweat is nothing we ever feel an urge to do. Once we have done it, however, we feel benefits promptly afterwards, which is why I urge you to get into the habit of making yourself get out of breath and sweat. Human beings are born to run, and we easily connect to a feeling that have supported our survival for thousands of years. You will notice that sooner than you think.

This fact means that the rewards from your training will come from your inside once you have started training.

Stick to 1K a day – and no more

The toughest thing about telling people about Couch Potato Fitness is the "fun" comments I get, such as "that's way too short to run" or "how can that make any difference."

I let people try it out.

And the reason that I have made it to my main task to broaden the knowledge about Couch Potato Fitness is that so many people have a (mis)understanding of training having to be very hard, to make a positive difference.

I have made it my mission in life to change the misunderstanding that running has to take long hours or be hard to make a positive difference!

It may sound like too much, to have to run every day, but if you stick to the plan (and not run more than I invite you to), you will not become overloaded.

One of my athletes, Bill, told me how the most important lesson he learned from me, happened during the first week of us working together. He had felt so good on his run that he ran 4K, and he was proud to have "over-performed."

Couch Potato Fitness is a rare example of a type of training, where you are not getting kudos for running farther than planned, and Bill remembers me saying "what is hard to understand about 1K?", which amused him.

After this day, Bill stuck to the program, and in his evaluation 4 months later, he told me that the most important lesson, he had learned was how much progress you could have, even when moving very slowly. Bill knew that without me as an accountability partner, he would have moved too fast, and most likely have injured himself – which he had tried several times before.

You may familiarize with like Bill, because many people share the trait of wanting to move forward fast, and thereby people train hard. Too hard.

> Remember that your obligation to your training will be to Couch Potato Fitness, and NOT to your own beliefs about how training should be done

I trained a man who first was very happy about the simplicity and short duration of the training, but after a few months, he felt strong enough to move things forward more than what the program prescribed. He insisted on running farther, and after the 15 weeks, he was injured, as he was not ready to run 3-4K a day only after 1½ months. I did not tell him "what did I say?", but what did I say?

> Let today be the first day in your new life with training! In other words, you have checked in, you have your boarding pass and on your way to the gate – ready for take-off!

As you are going to read about in the chapter Understanding The Psychology In Training, you have A LOT of reasons to NOT start training. If you lack motivation to start, trust that your motivation will appear during the first weeks.

One of the world's biggest apps for collecting data on physical activity, called Strava, elects the so-called "Quitter's Day" every year. Their data show, how the second Friday in January is the date, where most of the people, who started exercising on January 1st will quit. In other words, your New Year's resolution will last for approximately two weeks, unless you take all the challenges into account, which you will meet along your new way.

I hope that you reading these lines also means that you can commit yourself and start NOW.

The longer you wait, the farther away is your goal

When you are about to start, you could consider your replies to a few simple questions, that you see below. You can benefit from keeping your replies somewhere, for you to read again 15 weeks later. That is the simplest way of noticing your progress, once you have gotten well into Couch Potato Fitness.

And that's a promise!

You are NOT going to be able to remember what you expected or even hoped for once you have completed the training. Mainly because you have become a different person and will have set new goals by this time.

Keep it simple!

Write 1-2 sentences to each question, and keep them somewhere for you to read 15 weeks from now:

1. What do you want to get out of your training (mention a few areas of life)?
2. Describe a recurring problem, concerning yourself and your training
3. Write down – without thinking too much about it – what you see as the biggest challenge to reach the goal you have regarding training. And if you know why, you could write that as well.
4. What do you yourself think it takes for you to reach the goals you have set (at question no. 1 of this exercise)?

Take a photo of yourself

Your training starts on Day 1, and on that day, you take a photo of yourself – no shirt from the front and the side.

Pictures do not lie.

But remember to pose naturally, be honest with yourself and show what you look like today.

The purpose of seeing an image of yourself is to 1) see what status is, and 2) be able to follow the progress, you are making.

Keep the photo somewhere safe, and use it to check your starting point, and follow up along the way.

Look at your photo. Where are you on "The Pear Scale"?
(see the images below and compare)

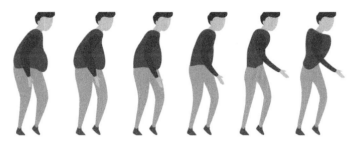

REMEMBER!

Seeing yourself with no clothes can be
a beautiful or horrific experience.

But do it anyway.

You will appreciate it soon.

I have been told how the Day 1 photo was used
as motivation, as already after a few weeks,
people were able to see the positive changes.

Do yourself a favor and follow your progression
with photos along the 15 weeks.

See yourself before your inner eye
How do you see yourself? And where do you wish to be?

Find some old photos of a fit you, where you have the body that you want.

With your vivid imagination, it is easy to see yourself on the screen of your mind.

The most amazing thing is that you can close your eyes, and see yourself pass the finish line as the winner of a big marathon!

Do not be shy to imagine big stuff.

☛ **Join the Facebook-group**
Couch Potato Fitness @onekayaday

Do not underestimate the benefits from sharing your experiences with like-minded. With or without a training partner (an accounta-bility partner), you get inspiration and can find support in our Facebook-group. You don't have to post or take part actively, but in this group, people are sharing their concerns as well as their victories. Here you can see a post from someone, who posted this photo as her first interaction with the group. Posts like this illustrate, what you can expect if you sign into

I have been out running every day for two weeks straight!

It has not been far, but I have tied those shoelaces in any weather, tired and on holiday. It has not at all been as bad as I thought it was going to be. Running used to be a big part of my life, but for the past 2 years it has been extremely difficult.

THANK YOU Christina for what you have inspired me to do, and thank you to everyone in this group who made a difference and inspired by posting.

I am gradually finding joy in running again.

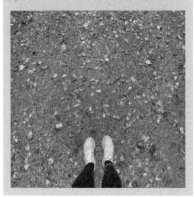

the group and let other people inspire and support you.

If you post yourself, you are likely to be an inspiration to others.

From now on you are an ATHLETE

Bill Bowerman was "the coach of all coaches," since he was the first of his kind, and he changed the world of running through his work. He was the head coach of the track & field team at University of Oregon for 24 years, and when he quit as a coach in 1973, he had been the coach of 16 of the 52 American runners, who – at that time – had ran sub 4 minutes on the mile (1.609 m).

IF YOU HAVE A BODY, YOU ARE AN ATHLETE
BILL BOWERMAN - COFOUNDER OF NIKE

Bowerman was a co-founder of Nike, and he is famous for saying that everyone with a body is an athlete. I love to use that expression about the people I coach. Therefore, from this day onwards, you are an athlete to me. And I invite you to get the same view about yourself.

See yourself as an athlete.

You are welcome to close your eyes and see yourself as someone who is light as the wind, who has a high energy level all through the day, and who is not physically limited in your daily life.

Spend a few minutes smiling because you are visualizing yourself as someone who gets up from the couch and takes the first step to becoming a stronger, healthier, more resilient, and happier version of yourself.

See yourself as the athlete, that you are.

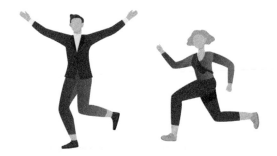

Understanding The Psychology In Training

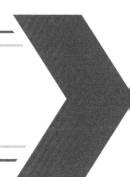

If you want the most important message from this whole chapter in one sentence, this is it; <u>your mindset is the most important thing to change</u>. And your mindset will be the center of attention to change during Couch Potato Fitness.

But before I will get into the details about your mindset and psychology, let us start with a wonderful story about a runner I admire much.

Casper Wakefield from Denmark holds the record

As a Dane, I am proud to share a world record of the toughest ultra-marathon Yucon Arctic Ultra, a 688-kilometer race, run in Canada, when the winter is at its worse with Casper Wakefield. I have had the pleasure of hearing Casper's catchy talk about his preparations and completion of that race. Casper was running for 7 days straight, he slept on average 2 hours a day during those 7 days. This was the first time I heard someone say, that mindset means 80% of your performance. Back then, I did not relate well, as I had mainly focused on preparing physically.

You do not have to run far distances to make use of the 80%-rule. My personal realization came after my mental breakdown in 2018. That was when I learned what it felt like to be mentally drained, and how being low on battery felt.

In 2018 I learned what it felt like to give up in advance. Until that time, I had always had energy levels high enough to get myself to stay in – at least some kind of – good physical shape.

The combination of my mental breakdown and all the years of experience with training, I now really understood what he meant. Unfortunately, only few personal trainers know how to exercise the mindset.

Casper generously shares his experiences on being prepared physically and with equipment to inspire and support other runners, and especially ultramarathon-runners. As part of his preparations, he would train in the coldest part of Sweden at his father-in-law's house, pulling car tires on ice, to adapt to running with a pulk. He analyzed and optimized his sleep patterns, and he also inspired me how to make space for all the (very) long runs, he also needed, while being a working dad in a family with three children.

I remember a great example of a family birthday, where he would run the 45K, and let the rest of the family arrive by car. This made the entire family happy and ready to be present at the birthday and not worry about getting home to do the training (I figure you can also eat a lot more cake, if you have just ran 45K!). That way Casper found many ways of combining family life with scary long runs. He was a huge inspiration to me!

Your mindset decides if you have given up in advance. I have not yet seen another training program with a focus on step-by-step guidance in 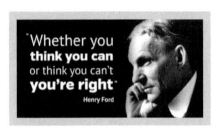 changing the 80% which has to do with the mindset.

Your mindset and your psychology is the root of your training. When your mindset is fit-for-fight to get you moving, you will be training with great ease. And if your mindset is programmed to NOT train – well, that is how it is going to be.

The most important "muscle" you have to exercise to get in better shape is the one placed between your ears. The program you are reading about in this book changes the fitness level of that important "muscle", as it will make physical training much more accessible and thereby possible.

The physical training in Couch Potato Fitness is so manageable, as this is the only way to change your habits around training.

Small steps. Again, and again.
The reason for me making training so simple is that it is very hard for people to take the first step. Training is something we humans do NOT prefer. Humans seek food, rest, and mating. Small insights into your genetic history will help you make it through all the psychological barriers that will arise, once you set your mind to persistent training. Following Couch Potato Fitness will give you all the necessary tools to avoid the many challenges, nature has installed in you.

This is the reason Couch Potato Fitness is so effective.

You are fighting an elephant!
Human beings have more than 50,000 years of genetic adaptation, and behavioral programming in only being physically active when we are escaping danger, or on a hunt. Food security and safety has only been a reality in the industrialized world during the past generation. Human beings save up for lean times, which means that as soon as we get the chance, we are most prone to eating and being lazy.

Picture how you are fighting an elephant because you are up against 50,000 years of evolutionary history, since your ancestors have always had a sharp focus on saving energy whenever possible and preparing for lean and dangerous times. Unfortunately, this genetic programming has created an overconsumption of food, and a sedentary lifestyle, which in turn has led to many of the lifestyle-related diseases we are struggling with: overweight, diabetes, high blood pressure and increased levels of blood fats, which are all contributing causes of premature deaths.

As soon as you become aware that your built-in laziness is genetic, and not part of your attitude, you can be happy to know that your mission on becoming more physically active has a profound resistance to it from yourself as well. In other words, you have a primordial power the size of an elephant, pulling in the opposite direction, when you are trying to get up from the couch – and this is the main reason why, getting up from the couch is a tough lift. You are heavier than an elephant!

The unknown makes habit changes so difficult

Another aspect of your psychology that is valuable to familiarize yourself with, is that habit changes are un-natural to us. It is easy to imagine how things are now, and we need help from someone outside, to be able to change the current habits.

The first good news is that you are reading this book. It means that you are interested in changing your habitual behavior. If you and I sat together, and I asked you about your dream-scenario regarding training, you would most likely start out by telling me why you had NOT done much about it already.

I have heard hundreds (literally!) of explanations to why people did not change their behavior themselves, so you are not alone. Most of the ones I meet, tell me in advance why daily training will be difficult to them. You are probably thinking that you are never going to train every day.

And for sure not with a smile on your face.

Never say never.

Human beings stick to habits for a feeling of security in the familiar. Security and predictability are key components of survival. We would not function as human beings if we woke up in a new place every day, go to a new job or hang out with new people. Therefore, to save energy and resources, we build up habits. Habits are healthy and good to have!

However, sometimes we stick to habits that are inappropriate, and we want to change them. If you think of the early days of Covid-lockdown, it was extremely hard to change the daily behaviors, but as soon as we had changed our behaviors, it was inconvenient to return to the habits we had before lockdown, right?

Habits are good to have around daily routines, and nice traditions around Christmas and birthdays, but whenever you want to change a habit, you must expect it to be hard work.

Let me comfort you that with Couch Potato Fitness habit changes happen in such small steps, and with consideration to the importance of small steps – that you will change your habit without you feeling it as hard.

When every step you must take is small, the task is manageable. Training that lasts for less than 10 minutes is manageable, and when you must train every day – no argument is necessary. You just do it.

The importance of smaller steps

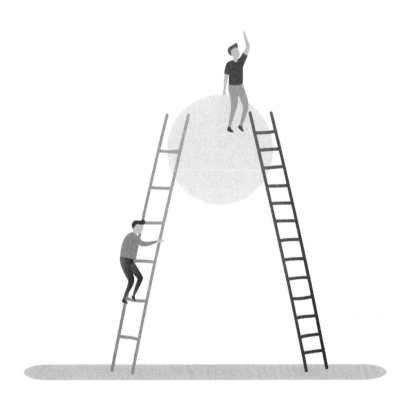

As you will learn all about in the chapter Onekayaday, Couch Potato Fitness is a daily workout, and the main reason for you maintaining five or more weekly trainings is for you NOT to have to argue with yourself whether you are training today.

Because whenever you start that argument, it most likely results in no training.

That goes for me too!

Couch Potato Fitness is not just something I am trying to "sell" to my surroundings. It is how I have trained since late 2019, and I am just sharing some honesties on how training works best.

I will let some of my former athletes explain the mechanism. Because all my athletes have changed their views on training. They are "telling a different story" now. The sooner you accept that training is not static, the better. Training is both something you can VIEW differently, and it can FEEL different from day to day.

The physical experience you will get from Couch Potato Fitness is just a fraction of what the training consists of. What it specifically will mean to you, is something you must discover as you go along.

Karsten told about his higher sense of self-worth, and a whole new discovery of what his body was capable of. Oskar no longer spent hours getting ready and changing into running clothes. And despite long working days and many obligations at work, Brian learned many new ways of incorporating training into his busy day.

Couch Potato Fitness is a process of training split up in such small tasks, that the habit change happens while you focus on solving a task split up in many small tasks.

"Small" tasks meaning that they are neither time consuming nor physically overwhelming to complete.

Every day.

And after 30 days you change the small task to be a-bit-bigger-but-still-very-small task every day.

Before you have completed even the first 30-day challenge, you will have experienced a huge change.

Couch Potato Fitness starts up taking 15 weeks, which is just something I have decided. Some studies show that habit change takes 21 days, while others point to the importance of staying in the new habit for up to ½ year before claiming the new habit set. The truth is somewhere in between. The most important thing is that you complete the three levels, that I have proposed.

You can experience a huge success taking up to one year completing the three levels – even the attempt to make your way through them will create a stronger and healthier you.

Just be patient. And trust what you read in this book.

Claim Your New Love:
Your Body

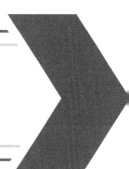

I have already invited you to think and speak about yourself as "an athlete". Most people, I have coached, laugh the first time I tell them to. A few have even rejected me, saying something in the line of "I will never become an athlete".

According to Bowerman's definition, you are an athlete! I will take my argument as far as claiming that the reason you (may) have had problems being consistent with your training IS that you think poorly about your body.

Let your participation in Couch Potato Fitness be associated with a newfound happiness about your body.

It is a choice to appreciate our bodies, and no matter how you do it, I would just recommend you do it MORE.

For what it's worth, your body has carried you around for your entire life. Your body is the amazing holster, which has made all your physical experiences possible. Fortunately, the body does not need daily appreciation to continue the "work" it does with keeping you upright and active. A short but daily appreciation from you recognizing what an amazing tool, your body is, will support your new self-image, and you will feel this in your performance.

I am happy to admit how I was talking to my legs on the night before my first final in a sprint meeting. I was running the finals at my very first competition, which was a 2 x 30 meters at an indoor youth championship, and I was trying to prepare myself the best that I could.

I won my first gold medal the day after.

I can tell you that all the greatest athletes see their bodies as unique and priceless machines, appreciated in both thoughts, words, and actions. All athletes take care of their bodies, and you are now invited to take part in this appreciation of human bodies.

In addition, many of my athletes have described to me how their self-worth and self-appreciation have gone up because they realize that their bodies have many more abilities, than what they had thought. Kevin described a newfound appreciation of his body in the evaluation he did after 15 weeks working with me. He told me about several pleasures connected with his newfound body appreciation. Apart from his weight loss and a normalized blood pressure, that he had struggled with being too high for several years, he felt proud. His body had become stronger, and he had increased the limits of what he had seen himself capable of. Kevin was also happy about his improved sex life, which he attributed to his greater joy about his body. Since there is a close connection between joy (and perseverance!) in our bodies having sex, I just want to invite you into a place, where you start ENJOYING everything about the body, you have.

You are hereby invited to be HAPPIER about your body and become familiar to appreciating it regularly.

Not only when your body is carrying you on your daily runs, but also when it is helping you around all day, to everything you choose to do on that day.

Another athlete of mine, Emily, described to me how her sleep had become much better, and how she felt her body calmer and more balanced. Sleep and sex are important ingredients to quality of life, and both are focused on your body.

We tend to think of our bodies as a tool that must work; we tend to complain about it when it does not work, but forget to praise it, when it does work. As you have already learned about in the importance of psychology in training, your mindset is crucial for your success.

There are many ways of praising your body, and you can do it right in lots of ways from now on. The only thing completely forbidden is to speak negatively about yourself or your body! What you do apart from that is up to you.

During the day, you are welcome to remind yourself, how happy you are about your body, and if you want to make big changes, find yourself some of the many meditations, available online (so-called "body scans"), that I will recommend you try. While contemplating and focusing on your body with an audio track, you can use your vivid imagination to see all the great changes about to happen to your physical and mental fitness level.

All great achievements are first seen with the mind's eye, so make sure that you focus on this part of your training as often as you can find the time to do it. Once a day is better than once a week, and once a week is better than once a month. You deserve it.

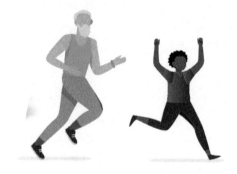

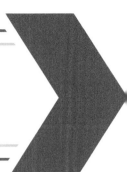

How You Overcome All The Excuses

Do not let the excuses stop you

I know you are busy. The day is full of to dos, and you do not know how to find the time to get your training done.

I expect you have many excuses since you have not done your training in the past. A typical excuse / objection / explanation is that you do not have time. That is what I have heard most times.

And I trust you have other excuses too.

Listen!! Your excuses have nothing to do with your training. Before we go into depth with the excuses, you need to:

Meet Benjamin who let his excuses stop him from training

Benjamin taught me how big a role excuses can play for our training. I met Benjamin in a work relation, and when he learned that I was a personal trainer, he became interested in trying out the training. Benjamin felt motivated to improve his own physical fitness, to become a stronger man at old age, than what he saw older men around him were.

During our first conversation, I told him the simplicity of Couch Potato Fitness and Benjamin immediately told me that he did not believe that such short duration of training would make significant changes. He continued to express his motivation to achieve the same good results he had heard about from my other athletes, and we agreed that he should start. But it took four weeks before he ran his first 1K.

Benjamin's own explanation to why it took that long, was that he had been on vacation, that his son was away for football-camp, and that he had had some busy weeks at work. During the first two weeks, he had five runs done. Every time we spoke, he would suggest alternatives to the running, such as playing soccer or hiking (what he already did).

After two months, he had reached a streak of 12 days with 1K a day, and on the 100 days of working with me, he had 30 1K's done. Even though I have never been able to understand why some people make up many excuses to avoid training, I understand the mechanisms from the psychology, and I am sorry to observe how "efficiently" all the excuses stop people from getting something done, that they really want to do.

Every time we spoke, Benjamin expressed a genuine wish to change his behavior, and become more fit. He never succeeded due to all the obstacles he laid out for himself. When we evaluated our training together, his own conclusion was that he had never been good at "doing what he was told." He had a more profound objection, which he had told me from the very beginning, that 1K a day would not make any difference.

He also evaluated that since he was in such (relatively) good shape compared to his peers, he did not feel much motivation after all.

Benjamin's skepticism and many objections efficiently ruined his chances of success.

When I reminded him that his original wish was to improve his physical fitness, and that he wanted to make a long-term contribution to his life and as an elderly man, his only comment was that he was actually in quite good shape.

This way, Benjamin really proved to me how human beings could do things short term that jeopardizes what they are REALLY wanting on a longer term. And unless we are directly affected, we are hesitant to exercise. (Much more about that in the chapter about Psychology).

The decision makes the difference – but it is only the first step!

Let's presume that you have made the decision that you do not have the time to train. In general, you are looking at it this way; you are not able to train, and you make up many explanations to why that is. In other words, you are deciding, that you do not have time. Moreover, the consequence is that you do not get your training done.

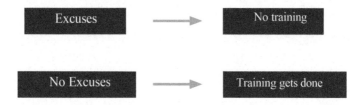

To turn this around, you could decide right now (as in RIGHT NOW!) that you are no longer going to listen to all your explanations to why you are not getting the training done – and then you will get it done!

You can change your behavior and have time for the training you want to do, and the way you do this, is as simple as finding 10-15 minutes every day, and complete your daily workout, which will change your thought patterns.

If you REALLY struggle with finding 10-15 minutes every day, you can do the exercise at the end of this chapter and ANALYZE YOUR DAY. You do this by checking your calendar and finding time to do your training instead of tasks that are less important than your training. Human beings DO NOT have time to do all the things we hope to do, and it is a subtle art, to remove what is – relatively – less important. Typical pitfalls are time spent on social media (could you make this 15 minutes less?), waiting time (e.g., when you attend your children's sports) or maybe you could just get up 20 minutes earlier than usual.

When you have decided to make space for your training, it means that something else must be removed. And hand on heart, your training should be one of the Top 2 things, you find time to do.

Now is the time for you to prioritize your own health and make your life longer and better at the end.

I know that it takes practice to find time for your daily run! And therefore, you just must … quiet your inner voice. That is the best start.

Tie your shoes. Shut yourself up. And get moving.

The many excuses all have the same solution!

Lack of time is the most common excuse to why training is postponed. You will find a specific solution to that at the end of the chapter.

Another typical excuse is the weather. That excuse can be used, if it is too hot or too cold. You may also have had a tough day at work. Or you think that you are not the kind of person, who will benefit from training every day. Or you are not up for the workload. Or you have a cold. Or you have slept poorly. Or you had one beer too many over lunch. Or you have caught a virus, and it may be dangerous to train. Or your legs may cramp. Or the body is sore from the training, and it will result in injuries to train. Or the kids are in a bad mood, and it is not a good idea to leave. Or that the partner is in a bad mood, and it is not a good idea to leave.

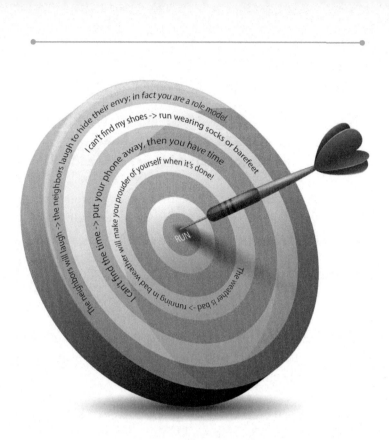

The neighbors will laugh -> the neighbors laugh to hide their envy; in fact you are a role model

I can't find my shoes -> run wearing socks or barefeet

I can't find the time -> put your phone away, then you have time

I can't find the time -> running in bad weather will make you prouder of yourself when it's done!

The weather is bad -> running in bad weather

RUN

All the excuses mentioned are just a sample of the excuses I have been told from people whom I have worked with.

And if you are ever in doubt, where to go for your run, because you find the area around your house un-inspiring, I will introduce you to Tim Franklin from Australia, who – during Covid-lockdown – ran a marathon inside his apartment. He was running laps of 21 meters, which he ran 2.010 times, finishing a marathon in 6 hours and 46 minutes.

All the excuses you see above have served a purpose when being mentioned, and you are welcome to add to the list with YOUR excuses. I invite you to make a long list of excuses!

It serves a purpose to drain all your frustrations by making up excuses. But do not let the excuses stop you from getting the training done!! In other words, NOW is the time for you to detach your training from all the excuses you make up and realize how ridiculous it is to both want to start training, and at the same time, talk yourself out of starting.

You HAVE already decided that you want more training in your life, so now you must be good to yourself and listen to your own decision.

If you do not experience excuses from getting your training done, you can skip to the next chapter of this book. But if you need a helping hand, you find that in the upcoming few pages. Here I deliver a few specific tools for inspiration, which can support you to set your priorities straight.

At the end of this chapter is a specific tool I use myself, every time I have lost track of my priorities around time especially in a busy period, or if I must make space for something new in my life.

This is something you want, so you must be good to yourself!

You must remember that your energy levels and self-discipline change during the day, and self-discipline is highest in the morning, and lowest in the evening. That is the simple reason to why you set out to get something done in the morning, which you will NOT get done at night or even in the afternoon. You must practice getting things done later in the day, so you must create a support system that can help you get (sh)it done, when your system calls for being lazy or impulsive at night.

It takes practice to follow your priorities and stick to the plans you are making with the most important person in your life – and that is you, of course.

☛ **The template on the next page can also be found www.couchpotatofitness.org**

Make time for the most important – by analyzing and prioritizing your day

Every time you are uncertain about your list of priorities in your own life, you should fill out the list below. The exercise seems simple but is very powerful to do. Remember to explain to yourself WHY the chosen areas are important. This will make it easier for you to plan your day and feel happy about your planning.

Prioritize your health, your family (maybe partner and children as two different points), your job, your home and your leisure time activities (what is most important to you, but find the 3-6 most important to you).

Prioritize what is most important to you:

My first priority is _____
because _____
My second priority is _____
because _____
My third priority is _____
because _____
My fourth priority is _____
because _____
My fifth priority is _____
because _____

Now you have a list of the five most important things in your life.

Then it is time to analyze your day. You choose two random days, and with the help of your calendar (and memory), you mark in your calendar when you spent time on the areas 1 to 5 in the above.

Next thing is to make an honest answer to the question whether your time spent is in accordance to your priorities? Are you spending most time on 1? And second-most time on 2? And third-most on 3…? You are getting the point. If not, now is the time to re-schedule. And plan. You allocate time to experience more of the 5 most important areas of your life.

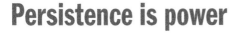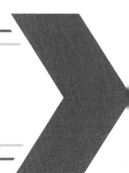

Persistence is power

Couch Potato Fitness will change your life A LITTLE BIT and your body A LOT.

The training program I am about to describe to you is a huge challenge. Not physically, but on many other levels.

The main challenge in the program is going to be psychological as the changes I invite you to do, are minor. The key to success is PERSISTENCE.

Because the training is very far from everything, you know about training already, and far from what "people" do when they want to get in shape.

It will therefore be a great advantage to you, if you wipe the board clean of everything else you know about training, and decide to trust me.

I am not able to explain to you why "people" think that training must be hard to make positive changes, or why "people" do not think that running 1K a day, can make a difference. I have always known that persistence pays off, and that small changes make a big difference in the long run. And this is the principle of Couch Potato Fitness.

Apart from the psychological challenge of moving slower than you are used to, being persistent is another challenge. You must do something every day. But what you must do, takes such short time, that it is hard not to do. You will be successful if you do what is described on the following pages.

Throughout the book, you are guided to the training, the program, good ways to start up, the excuses and the psychology in training.

You will be well prepared for the challenges you are going to meet.

But above all you have to be comfortable with being persistent.

With those words, it is time to go through what it is all about.

Onekayaday

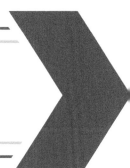

Couch Potato Fitness is 1K a day

Couch Potato Fitness is a training program in three levels.

To start at Level 1, all you need is a pair of running shoes, that you can put on and run 200-300 meters in.

The program starts at Level 1, and you are allowed and ready to proceed to Level 2, WHEN YOU HAVE COMPLETED LEVEL 1.

And you are allowed to proceed to Level 3 WHEN YOU HAVE COMPLETED Level 2.

It is simple, but not easy.

Each level contains comprehensive learning, and if you skip a level, you can expect to achieve less than the full result.

For each level I know that you will be able to achieve more and more both metaphorically and literally speaking, and

I also expect that you will maintain and even enjoy the lifestyle as a couch potato, which is why the name seemed appropriate.

Couch Potato Fitness is planned to last for 15 weeks. Or 105 days. Getting through the habit changes in three levels will take this time, and it is an appropriate time span for lasting lifestyle changes to occur.

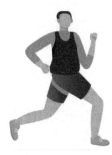

Level 1 is to complete a 30-day streak[1] of running 1K every day. That's all! You are probably already hearing an inner voice telling you that this is not a good way of training, but I invite you to try it out anyway.

Trust me

Simply put, Level 1 is that you spend 10 minutes every day for 30 consecutive days, challenging your joints, bones, and ligaments, and do something that makes you sweat. And this is done best by running 1K. If you are ABSOLUTELY incontrollable, and you are used to

---

[1] *A "streak" is from sports, when a team has continuous wins, a winning streak*

running already, and want to run farther, the maximum allowed distance in Level 1 is 2K (a day).

If you skip a day, all you must do is to start over. For example, if you have run 1K for 17 consecutive days, and miss Day 18, this is a new Day 0, and the next Day 1 will be as soon as you start again.

Starting again is simple. The course is clear, and there is no need to feel ashamed about missing a day in your streak. Just get back on track. I have no clue to how many times I have started again, and given myself a new Day 1, and my excellent physical shape is due to my skill of just starting again as soon as possible.

Just do it.

In a perfect world, you are completing Level 1 during the first 30 days, you continue into Level 2 for another 30 days, and then you can continue for 4-6 weeks on Level 3. In this way you will experience an immense habit change, while you are counting days on the different levels.

Once you are on Level 3, you have got training as part of your daily life.

Real life experiences are that only 1 out of 6 complete Level 1 during the first 30 days. Like I said in my introduction; it is simple, but not easy.

EVERYONE, who starts at Level 1, experience benefits from the habit change and the altered lifestyle, since there is immediate positive feedback to be felt both in the body and mind.

Since focus is purely on doing a bit of training, that ONLY takes 10 minutes per day, the discussion with oneself about whether to get on with it, is minimized or maybe even eliminated – which is totally new to many people.

Regardless of how many times it will take you to complete Level 1, a new Day 1 is another great step towards completing Level 1 – and thereby feeling the reward in getting closer to the next level.

And remember; it is a greater success to work on completing level 1 for a year, than to skip training altogether, because you feel bad about starting over for the 10th time.

Just do it.

Keep on running.

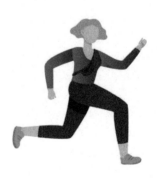

LEVEL 1: START-UP AND HABIT CHANGE

➢ **START-UP:** You declare your Day 1 by taking a photo of yourself, as naked as you feel comfortable, cut away your head in the photo and take two, one from the front and one from the side. See page 75 for more details on a good start in the chapter "All You Need".

➢ **DAY 1 TO 30:** You do a daily run of 1-2K. Daily. As in EVERY DAY. Preferably 1K. If you are not able to run 1K without stopping, you run for as long as you can, and then you walk 100 steps. Count out loud while walking. And then you run again until you cannot run any more, and walk for 100 steps, counting your steps. Occupy your mind with counting your steps.

Remember to track your runs (use e.g. Nike Run Club / NRC, an excellent free app for both iPhone and Android). A large part of your training is that you can look back and see what you have achieved, which makes it very important, that you log your activities.

There are lots of available digital resources, and you just find the one, that is most appropriate to you.

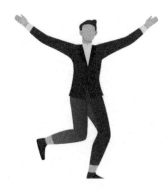

Your Day 1 photo is a good start, and you are welcome to monitor your progression this way, by taking photos with 2-3 weeks in between. Pictures don't lie.

Level 2: MAINTENANCE

> **Level 2** is another 30-day challenge that starts immediately after Level 1 is complete.

> Day 31 in Level 1 is also Day 1 on Level 2.

On Level 2 you run 1.3 times the number of kilometers you ran (on average) at Level 1. In other words, if you ran 1K a day on Level 1, you are allowed to run 1.3K on Level 2. And if you ran 1½K a day on Level 1, you are allowed to run 2K a day in your Level 2 streak.

Level 3: MAINTENANCE AT A WEEKLY BASIS

> ➤ **Level 3** is counted at a weekly basis, where you train 5 or more times a week. The weekly target is 1.3 times the total number of kilometers completed at Level 2. In other words, if you ran 14K a week (2K a day) on Level 2, you run 18K on level 3. On Level 3 you count from Monday to Sunday, and you can distribute your runs as you prefer. Strive for >5 weekly trainings to keep momentum and avoid discussions with yourself about whether you should run. You can learn more about why this is important in the chapter "The Psychology In Training".

A necessary element is that you find yourself a partner to hold you accountable to. This way you will help each other to complete the three levels *(more about this in the chapter "All You Need")*

Now that you are familiar with what Couch Potato Fitness is all about, I want you to meet Ellen.

Meet Ellen, who started out to prove the program wrong

Ellen is a woman I know privately, and since I started talking about a training program based on running, she gave me fun comments that she was not "the running type", but also that she wanted to improve her shape.

She also wanted to find a type of training, that could benefit her two children, so that they could all get in better physical shape. I never tried to persuade her into trying out Couch Potato Fitness, but one day she declared, that she would try out "this running, that you always talk about".

She found her old running shoes (that I later realized were more than 20 years old, so that does not even have to be a barrier!), and she started out on her first 30-day challenge with 1K a day.

As most others Ellen noticed how the short distance made the task easily done and therefore feasible. She is part of the minority of 15-20% of my athletes, who completed Level 1 in their first attempt. Before she had completed Level 1, she was honestly puzzled about how fast the feeling of wellness had come to her, and how she looked forward to her daily 1K run.

Halfway through Level 2, Ellen experienced a sore knee, so she was not able to run for a few days. During those few days of not running, Ellen already sounded like an elite athlete, who was complaining about her not being able to train. She said "I miss running" followed by "OOOH MY GOD, I had never thought, I would say something like that!".

Ellen gave me a great example of the importance of keeping your streak, when she went to France (from Denmark) by car with her family.

In advance, she had expected that this trip would interrupt her streak, and that she would have to start over. (I would think that a 1K would be a perfect way to "stretch the body" after a whole day in a car, but I am 100 % aware, that I am different at this point).

In the evening, the family was in a small French town, looking for a hotel. Ellen had been dropped in front of a hotel, and her family was suddenly in a car 800 meters from her. She now had to walk to meet them and got the – in my opinion fabulous! – idea to run to them. So she grabbed her sandals in her hands, hugged her boobs and activated the running app on her first spontaneous run. When she reached the parking lot, she

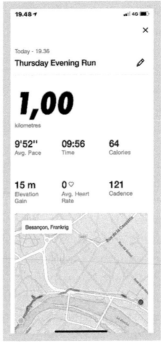

Ellens trackede løbetur, der rummer en skøn historie

had to take 5-6 rounds to reach the 1K. This is another way to get (sh)it done!

Stories like Ellen's tell me, what a solid program Couch Potato Fitness is. I am hoping that you feel like trying it out, so you can achieve your own positive experiences—and weird places to track your 1K!

To increase your motivation to get through Level 1 and Level 2, I have made a "diary" for you to print and post somewhere visible to you. Somewhere like your refrigerator door. The "diary" is just 30 blank squares on a piece of paper, but they will support you in holding yourself accountable, and follow your progress through Level 1.

And Level 2 after that.

Keeping a visual diary is a simple and effective way of sharing your training with the people you live with, or those who visit you. And it will be a reward to yourself every time you open the fridge door!

You can see an example of a diary in the end of this chapter. You can download it as pdf on www.couchpotatofitness.org

I cannot stress the importance of keeping track of your training enough. When keeping track, you create an important tool for yourself, that will motivate you already after a few days. Anyone who thinks, that 1K a day is "next to nothing", will during the first few weeks have run more than they have run for many months, or maybe even years. Keeping track will motivate and support you immensely.

But you need to experience this personally before you will believe me.

Let me share Mia's experience that she posted in the Facebook-group @onekayaday after only two weeks. Mia felt how the 1K run felt extremely hard to complete, and if it had not been for her tracking, she would not have noticed the reward!

As you can see in her post, Mia had improved by more than 1 minute over the first two weeks, even though the training only took 7 minutes to complete. No wonder the training felt hard, with such great improvements.

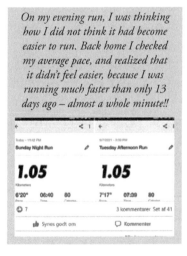

On my evening run, I was thinking how I did not think it had become easier to run. Back home I checked my average pace, and realized that it didn't feel easier, because I was running much faster than only 13 days ago – almost a whole minute!!

Training is always going to feel hard, and regardless if you're running 7m17s or 6m20s per kilometer, this is how it is supposed to be. In less than two weeks, Mia had improved so much, and if she had not had her tracking on her watch to tell her the difference in the data, she would have considered the "hard" run a defeat. Because of her tracking, it became a success. I sincerely hope that you will bring your mobile phone or watch every time, for you to track your run.

The template to print and post somewhere visible, on your bathroom mirror or refrigerator door, works well as motivation and a daily reminder every time you brush your teeth or open the fridge. All tricks apply!

As you will read about in the rest of this book, we as humans are NOT designed to change our habits, so all the little tricks you plan to make your habit change work, are important.

Gamification in Couch Potato Fitness

If you think that Level 1, Level 2 and Level 3 are something taken from gaming, you are right. As you will learn in this book, human biology and psychology are the foundation for our lack of ability to get our training done.

Much the same way, we have an inner need to be rewarded, and this need is satisfied when achieving new levels while working or playing a game. When at Level 1, I do not know what is available to me on Level 2, but I strive to achieve it anyway. A term known as gamification. I have added these elements to my program, and I expect you will feel the effect.

Your wish to achieve a 30-day streak speaks louder than all the excuses you can come up with, that tries to talk you out of changing your behavior.

As a post in the Facebook-group shows, it seems worth striving for. As stated by the person who posted his image of his Garmin app, it had been highly satisfactory to be able to take the screenshot and share it with his accountability partner.

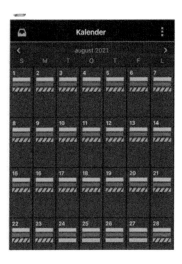

All apps used to encourage training are generous in the use of encouragements, awards, kudos, and tell you about all the records you are beating. Take everything you can get in this tough beginning!

Another advantage by using an app, is that you will get acquainted with the reactions from your body, starting to develop body awareness. Your habit change will be followed by major changes, both physically and psychologically. Especially in periods when your body is struggling, we tend to think, that it is best NOT to do a workout. Adding consistency to your training will teach you how your body will become more alive and fresher after a short workout, when you feel tired, than if you stay on the couch.

Injuries are what happens when we have trained too hard or have ignored body signals. But along the way, you will discover, that your new (increased) level of activity, will give you an excellent opportunity to better know your amazing body. In this process, you benefit immensely from tracking your training.

On the last page of this chapter, you can see a suggestion to the tracking I invite you to fill out. From day to day, you give yourself an overview of your training, including the small comments, you provide yourself daily.

Comments should relate to both the time of day of your training, the pace you kept and how it felt. Your app will note your pace in minutes and seconds, but the FEELING is something only you can register. And given that we all forget details about what happened 2-3 days ago, you need to take notes to yourself every day. A low-feeling day can immediately be followed by an up-turn (and vice-versa), so turning it into a habit to record the reactions from your body, will quickly increase your body awareness.

As you get to know your body even more, you will get into the habit of training, you will also get into the habit of appreciating how the body will "speak" to you even more (which you can read more about in the chapter "Claim Your New Love: Your Body").

During your reading of this book, you will learn why human beings are not easily activating themselves. You will attain an understanding of the mechanisms at play once you have read all the chapters. If you have JUST read the preceding chapter, and you now know that you should run every day, you may think of this as a big task.

As you have already learned (more) about, the task to change behavior IS daunting.

The following chapters will support your decision on making your lifestyle changes, and no worries; you have a Chinese proverb to support you in being patient.

THE BEST TIME TO PLANT A
TREE WAS 20 YEARS AGO

THE SECOND-BEST TIME IS NOW

CHINESE PROVERB

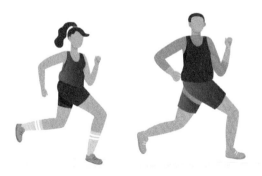

Level 1, day 1:	Level 1, day 2:	Level 1, day 3:	Level 1, day 4:	Level 1, day 5:
Ran 1.01K just before dinner and walked twice. OMG my legs hurt!	Ran 1.01K before breakfast. Three short walks, legs feeling better	Ran 1.03K with only one walk (yay!), just before breakfast (weekend)	Ran 1.00K with VERY sore legs. At 10 pm, just HAD to get it done!	Ran 1.05K while lasagna was in the oven, did not want a night-run again. Legs are better, but I walked three times.
Level 1, day 6:	Level 1, day 7:	Level 1, day 8:	Level 1, day 9:	Level 1, dagy10:
Ran 1.20K with only one walk, legs felt good, but now my knees are sore. Ran just before bedtime, which is not working, I can not sleep after.	Ran 1.00K with NO WALK! Very proud! My time was 7m30s, I ran just before I left from work, this worked well!	Ran a very long 1.10K, had had a Friday-beer at work, NOT GOOD TO RUN ON BEER!	Ran 1.00K before breakfast with the family, 7m1s, I want to break 7m tomorrow! Morning runs are better for me.	Ran 1.20K, it went well, 7m3s, I am looking too much at the watch. Got up early, maybe better during the day?

Level 1, day 11:	Level 1, day 12:	Level 1, day 13:	Level 1, day 14:	Level 1, dag 15: ...
Ran 1.10K, dressed in my running clothes taking A to swimming lessons, that was a great solution! Monday run from now on.	Ran 1.40K, what?!? It went so easy today, 6m50s, without me thinking about it! I ran while F picked up the girls.	Ran 1.15K, it is easier now, but the knees need a warmup, 7m2s.	Ran 1.25K in my lunch break. That works very well! 6m45s, the middle of the day is great for me	
Level 1, day 16:	Level 1, day 17:	Level 1, day 18:	Level 1, day 19:	Level 1, day 20: ....

Examples of how the registration can be done on (part of) Level 1. All from athletes on Level 1.

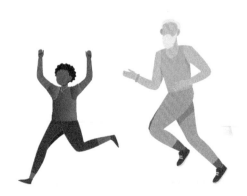

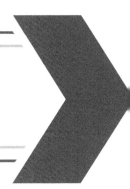

The Scientific Evidence

Scientific evidence can motivate even more

This book describes a training method, that targets everyone who wants to improve their physical and mental health, by being a (bit) more physically active.

Nevertheless, I have a favorite target group which are all male members of a population. The main reason is that men seem to be generally challenged when it comes to keeping a healthy level of physical activity. The most consistent finding within public health science is the inequality in health, between men and women.

Men have shorter life expectancy than women

Across the world, women become older than men in the same country, but it has not always been like this[2]. Until the 19th century, the higher mortality was found among women, which changed remarkably with the medical advances during the 20th century. After 1944, when penicillin was discovered, people no longer died from infectious diseases to the same extent, what had

---

[2]   *www.ourworldindata.org*

previously killed relatively more women in connection to child-birth.

Now the scenario in all countries around the world, is that women live longer than men. The difference is as little as ½ year in Bhutan, and as much as 11 years in Russia. In many countries, such as Denmark, an increased inequality between men and women has happened over the past 50 years, showing that the longevity of men has not improved as much as for women. One explanation is smoking. Historically speaking, men have smoked for longer, and much more than women.

The difference between women's and men's longevity is both due to behavior and psychology. Female hormones seem to protect from many lifestyle related diseases. Also, the natural storages of fat on women – around the waist and breasts – are causing less disease than the typical storages for men, in and around the belly, known as visceral fat. Many scientific sources have claimed that the "pear shape" of a man is the more dangerous body shape, since visceral fat is a risk factor to suffering from heart disease.

We die from cancer and heart disease, and the quality of life is affected negatively by diabetes In many developed countries such as my home-country Denmark and also the U.S., one third of the deaths in a human population are caused by heart disease, and another one-third die of cancer. The rest die from several other causes.

Diabetes – and poor mental health – affect the quality of life. There are two types of diabetes, Type 1 and Type 2, and Type 2 is the type you get later in life, typically due to a lifestyle of unhealthy diet and physical inactivity. In this chapter, I choose to focus on cancer, heart disease and diabetes, since these are all preventable diseases.

In other words, these are diseases you can prevent by changing your lifestyle, and thereby reduce your personal risk in obtaining.

Obesity, heart disease and cancer are public health diseases

Public health diseases are highly prevalent diseases.

In many countries around the world, obesity is prevalent among half of the adult population. Obesity causes several health problems, such as diabetes, impotence, and joint problems. It also makes other diseases worse, apart from affecting mental health which is lower among people that are overweight or obese.

Cancer has many causes, but overweight increases the risk of more than 13 different types of cancer[3].

In Denmark with around 6 million people, ¼ million people are living with Type 2-diabetes, and even among diabetics, women have better survival rate than men

_____

[3] *"Danskernes viden om og holdninger til overvægt og sundhed 2019" af Kræftens Bekæmpelse og Sundhedsstyrelsen, fundet på www. sundhedsstyrelsen.dk*

with diabetes[4]. This is partly due to the delayed response from men to their symptoms, and the fact that they generally hesitate to go see their doctor. This male trait of postponing to ask for help is known as the Tarzan Syndrome.

The risk of developing Type 2-diabetes increases with age, but during the later generations, younger people are hit, due to changed lifestyle with more physical inactivity, and increased prevalence of obesity. Type 2-diabetes is hereditary, so if anyone in your family has had it, it is an even better idea to get a medical check-up to determine if you have it – or you are at risk of getting it. Whether or not you get Type 2-diabetes relies mostly on your health behaviors, mainly your level of physical activity and your diet. If you are carrying "extra load" on your body, and it is placed around your stomach area, your risk of disease is even higher. Type 2-diabetes gives a high level of sugar in the blood, which – over time – wears out the nerves and blood vessels in your body.

When people with diabetes are treated, medical staff will monitor blood circulation, impaired vision, wounds (mainly on the feet) that will not heal, and impotence. Even though the treatment of Type 2-diabetes is medical, the disease can be treated with lifestyle changes. A higher level of physical activity and dietary changes can change blood sugar levels and reduce the risk of serious diseases that follow having Type 2-diabetes.

---

[4] *"Men's Health Week: Mænd og Type 2-diabetes", fra www.apotek.dk*

Sex is an important part of life

Overweight, heart disease and diabetes often affect sex life negatively. So the quality of your sex life can give you a hint about early stages of lifestyle related diseases, that are preventable by lifestyle changes. Impotence or erectile dysfunction becomes more common with age, and while 10% of 50-year-old men experience erectile dysfunction, this is common for 30-50% of men with diabetes at the same age.

To have a well-functioning sex life, you need well-functioning blood and nervous systems, which are both challenged among people with diabetes. Overweight, bad physical shape and smoking are causes that can be changed to improve your sex life.

The results from a Danish PhD-dissertation from 2021[5] which examined the association between physical activity and problems with the sex life, concluded that 3 hours of cardiovascular training per week was the optimal to improve erectile dysfunction[6]. Cardiovascular training will improve endurance during sex since the quality and duration of the erection depends on blood flow and muscular strength.

---

[5] *Helle Gerbild, "Physical activity to reduce vascular erectile dysfunction", Aalborg Universitet, 2021*

[6] *Gerbild H et al. "Physical activity to improve erectile dysfunction: A systematic review of intervention studies", Sexual Medicine 2018;6:75-89.*

In other words; if you – or someone close to you – experience problems in your sex life, you can expect improvements also in that area, when you have been through Couch Potato Fitness. Better physical condition and more muscles will improve performance both in- and outside the bedroom.

The purpose of the training described in this book is to give you a lifestyle with habits of consistent moderate physical activity, which will improve your physical condition and increase muscular capacity, with the benefit of getting slimmer along the way.

The collection of scientific evidence, studying the association between exercise and mortality, has consistently shown, that moderate levels, where you get out of breath and sweaty several times a week, is healthier than training very hard only a few times a week. Couch Potato Fitness also considers what has shown most effective to reduce overweight and cardiovascular disease and to improve mental health. Scientific evidence supports moderate physical activity 4 hours a week.

World Health Organization[1] (WHO) recommends that adults (aged 18+ years) should do at least 150–300 minutes of moderate-intensity aerobic physical activity; or at least 75–150 minutes of vigorous-intensity aerobic physical activity; or an equivalent combination of moderate- and vigorous-intensity activity throughout the week should also do muscle-strengthening activities at moderate or greater intensity that involve all major muscle groups on 2 or more days a week, as these provide additional health benefits.

May increase moderate-intensity aerobic physical activity to more than 300 minutes; or do more than 150 minutes of vigorous-intensity aerobic physical activity; or an equivalent combination of moderate- and vigorous-intensity activity throughout the week for additional health benefits. should limit the amount of time spent being sedentary.

Replacing sedentary time with physical activity of any intensity (including light intensity) provides health benefits, and to help reduce the detrimental effects of high levels of sedentary behaviour on health, all adults and older adults should aim to do more than the recommended levels of moderate- to vigorous-intensity physical activity.

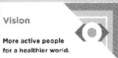

Vision

More active people for a healthier world.

Mission

To ensure that all people have access to safe and enabling environments and to diverse opportunities to be physically active in their daily lives, as a means of improving individual and community health and contributing to the social, cultural and economic development of all nations.

Target

A 15% relative reduction in the global prevalence of physical inactivity in adults and in adolescents by 2030.

---

[1] *World Health Organization Fact Sheet on physical activity, (-> Newsroom/Fact sheets/Detail/Physical activity)*

All you need!

The essential part of getting the work done!

You only need two things to get fit. This goes for every athlete on the planet, whether you are professional / elite or "just" someone getting back in shape after pregnancy, a busy period at work or whatever you have dealt with lately that made you a couch potato.

The two things you need are:

1) A plan
2) An accountability partner

The internet is loaded with plans on how to get fit.

(But none of the others are so simple as onekayaday, so just stick to that for now)

So the plan is the easiest part.

The crucial and most important aspect of following the plan, is that you have an accountability partner. Someone who knows what you are planning to do, and who follows up.

Ideally, your accountability partner is also a training partner, who has the same goal as you; to get fit.

But it surely does not have to. It can be someone from work, in your family or even a teenager around you, who would just be consistent and supportive to ask you about your daily workout.

As you read about in the chapter "Understanding The Psychology In Training" Couch Potato Fitness in essence is over a course of 15 weeks. This is a choice I have made from the academic knowledge I have on behavior change.

Some claim that a behavior is changed after 21 days, but ask a smoker about this…

Other studies say up to 90 days, and my experience with athletes, who believed they had changed their behavior after Level 1 / the first 30 days, is that you need to get further than Level 1. Somewhere between Level 2 and Level 3, you can expect the feeling of a new habit to have kicked in.

The most important thing for your success is that you complete the three levels whether this will take 2-3 times as long.

> **Three important pieces of advice on your training:**
>
> 1. get yourself a training partner
> 2. get yourself an accountability partner
> 3. team up with someone else

The fact is, that if you are only accountable to yourself, and have told no one else about your intentions with the training, you have a 10-15% chance of success. But if you share your goal with someone else, you have an 85-90% chance of success.

You can also just share your ambition on social media, and let your contacts know what your goal is. By just doing this simple act of saying it out loud, you will sense how the obligation will change your mindset.

The Healthy Lifestyle

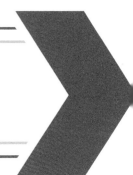

This is how you fuel your body

The physical condition of your body is basically the result of a balance between what you consume and what you burn. A book about training must therefore have a section about how you fuel your body, for optimal support in your everyday life, and to optimize your training.

I will begin by announcing that this chapter will have no restrictions or counting of calories.

On the contrary

You are likely to be surprised about my dietary recommendations. First and foremost, I invite you to be more mindful of the way you fuel your body. If you follow all the recommendations in this chapter, you are going to experience a body, very ready for the training, you are going to ask from it. Secondly, you will experience to thrive more in general.

Before I tell you how you can fuel your body optimally, I want you to meet Michael:

Meet Michael – who now ENJOYS his bacon

I am introducing to you Michael, who took 30 years to learn that he was fully capable of running. Michael experienced some remarkable changes when I introduced Couch Potato Fitness to him. It may have been his positive attitude that attributed to the success he experienced, because before he started running, he would have sworn that he could be a person, who would enjoy a run.

I met Michael close to his 50th birthday, and he was feeling low since several friends his own age had gotten life-style related diseases, and he felt them coming closer. Michael had worked to improve his health for many years, but his effort had often resulted in frustration and "yo-yo-weight", as the programs he followed had not resulted in long-term effects maintained. He was sad when we started working together.

Michael owns his own company together with two friends and colleagues. Michael's mindset BEFORE we started working together was that he had had many different attempts to change his health behavior, he had lost weight several times (and gained it again), and always thought he would never be able to run, after some serious knee-injuries at the age of 19. Michael is a former elite-level badminton-player, and he vividly remembers how it felt to be in good shape, and for many years he had missed the joy of training.

Michael learned from Couch Potato Fitness that his body is still very quick at adapting to the moderate level of physical activity, and his craving after sweets and fast-food changed.

I was amused when he called me and told me that the pizza he shared with some friends tasted like cardboard-paper!

I believe that your tastebuds also change when you get in a better shape. Michael experienced a changed attitude towards his diet, and a broader perspective on what healthy lifestyle was, after he learned what you are about to hear about in this chapter.

Couch Potato Fitness taught Michael a new, healthy lifestyle that surprised him. He was convinced that he was not able to run, but after a few gentle encouragements, he finally agreed to try a 1K with walking included. The first 3-4 weeks he told me how he was afraid that his knees might break (those were his words!), but after being persistent, he gradually felt how his body became stronger and – more importantly – how the fear gradually left him, and he started to enjoy the daily runs.

Prior to Couch Potato Fitness Michael had spent a few hours every day on walking, this being his physical activity, and even though he still enjoys his walks, part of the purpose with Couch Potato Fitness is that your training is completed in a very short time.

The "dietary recommendations" you also get in this chapter opened Michael's eyes to further perspectives on diet and to what a healthy lifestyle also is – and that your sleep pattern and intake of water are important parts of a healthy lifestyle. Thus, the food you eat is less important than getting all the other components in place.

Michael's biggest surprise was that he is now able to enjoy his bacon without feeling guilty or unhealthy, because intake of fats/sugar/salt has very little to do with your body being strong and healthy. Now we share the joke that bacon IS a vegetable.

I have been SO happy to learn about Michael's genuine joy over his lifestyle changes because he tells me that he knows that Couch Potato Fitness is the type of lifestyle change that will keep him fit for the rest of his life. He has told me this with his typical big smile on his face. During our training together, he hurt his foot and could not run for several weeks. Saying "I miss running" was NOT words that Michael would have thought would come out of his mouth, but this shows what Couch Potato Fitness can do to people.

As the very first thing, Michael and I would go through his health behavior, as this was what he felt most urgent to deal with, when wanting to improve his health. My best advice to improve your health behavior is what you find in this chapter. I started by asking him the subtitle of the chapter; how do you fuel your body?

My starting point when I talk to people about diet and health related lifestyle is very far from public dietary recommendations. My approach is very tangible and specific, as it is focusing on the most necessary "fuels", our body needs. I think that most people fail to recognize that oxygen and water are the most important ingredients for staying alive.

Humans die after 3 minutes with no air, and 3 days with no water. The rule of thumbs is 3 weeks with no food, so bear in mind that you can survive long without food, which should tell you, that the food is not the most important aspect of your health.

In my humble opinion, the food you eat is only the 4th most important ingredient. Because I rate sleep as such an important part of a healthy lifestyle, which most people tend to ignore.

My 1st piece of advice: AIR

The most important part of your body's energy level is the air you breathe. You breathe 20,000 times a day, without even thinking about it (pssst, your amazing body does that without you doing anything, isn't that cool??)

So many places in the health business, and in relation to stress-relief, mindfulness, and yoga, it is pointed out how important our breathing is to us. I just hope you will become more aware of your breathing from now on. I invite you to "only" do 200 deep breaths every day, and make them in through your nose, or "just" as deep as you can, and then notice what happens in your body, while doing this.

You can do your breathing exercise from anywhere you are. Somewhere sitting on a park bench or in your car, and you can breathe in (through your nose, which increases the healthy nitrogen oxide), and slowly breathe out through your mouth.

If you do 10-20 breathings, you will not only calm your heart, your mood, and your pulse, but you will immediately get clearer thoughts. Breathing deeper, will increase your level of oxygen, you will think better, and make sharper decisions while oxygenating all cells in your body.

During your runs it is essential that you breathe deeply, and it will always be an advantage to your body to pay attention to your breathing at a general level.

If you are interested in more information about the healing effects of your breathing, I invite you to start following the Danish world record holder in free diving, Stig Severinsen. I also recommend you find Wim Hof and his method and take one of his (free) online classes. He can teach you a unique method to ventilating your body, which will increase your energy level spontaneously. Wim Hof (The Ice Man) is a phenomenon, who has climbed Mt Everest with very little clothes on. Even though he appears like a person from another planet, his teaching in breathing exercises is so tangible, that I will recommend you spend the few minutes it takes, to go through his master class.

> **How often are you mindful about breathing deeply?**
>
> The recommendation to improved health is to give yourself (at least) 200 deep breaths every day

My 2nd piece of advice: WATER

The second most important factor to the energy level of your body is water. Liquid is important to maintain bodily functions, and our bodies consist of approximately 60% water. Given that we secrete 1-2 liters every day, it is crucial to add water. If you have been physically active or been ill (felt sick or sweated a lot) you have lost more than average water. The need for liquids varies between people, but a normal recommendation is to drink 1-2 liters of water every day. Preferably water or other liquids with no sugar or alcohol.

How much do you drink every day?

Recommended for optimal health is to
drink at least 2 liters of water every day
(with a twist of lemon or bubbled water)

My 3rd piece of advice: SLEEP

The next important thing to maintain a healthy level of energy is to regenerate during sleep.

Sleep is a necessity to all living creatures, and the lack of sleep will affect both the immune and hormonal system, and your memory and learning skills directly. If you have children, you know the immediate effects of mood and thriving, when you are without your sleep for shorter or longer.

The three times I have been on maternity leave, I have experienced periods of several months, where I did not sleep for more than 3-4 hours straight, and during those times, I was often thinking how sleep depriving is a method used as torture. And I could relate well! It is noticeable on the body and mind, and I find it thought provoking, that so many people exercise "self-torture" by going to bed after midnight and getting up a few hours later. There are plenty of studies on the negative health effects of night-shift workers, and this is another reason to stress the importance of good sleep habits if wanting to stay healthy.

Sleep is a huge research area, and we all seem to know, that 7-8 hours of sleep and steady habits are healthy to us.

It is not only the duration of your sleep that plays a role, but also WHEN you sleep. Your body has a natural preference to sleep around midnight, and you may know this, if you have had periods where you went to bed a few hours before midnight. You will then feel much more rested. I often notice the truth in an advice I got from a midwife, to sleep before midnight, because every 1 hour of sleep I got this time of the night would count for 2. The body responds immediately on your choice of bedtime, as you feel if you decide to stay up until midnight. Suddenly you feel fresher, and this is your body's way of responding to the "fight-mechanism" in us all; the body believes that you are the one staying up all night to guard the group in the cave and gives you hormonal kicks to stay awake.

Otherwise, you would have gone to bed several hours earlier.

This mechanism is not healthy for us on a longer term, as the excretion of stress hormones wears down our bodies. Also, if you want to release some fat, your body will not allow this, since it is not clever to lose fat when in danger. So, if you wish to lose weight, your sleep patterns are extremely important.

How many and from what time do you sleep at night?

Recommended for optimal health is to sleep at least 7 hours every night, and always between 11 pm and 1 am, that are the most important hours to regenerate your body.

My 4th piece of advice: FOOD

The next thing our bodies need, are the nutrients you get from what we eat.

Food is a cultural thing, and even what is considered "healthy" is – in my opinion – a cultural thing. Your eating habits are characterized by where in the world you come from, and the family you grew up in, and from all of this, you have created your own culture around the foods you eat.

I am not going to educate you on what is good for you because you know this yourself.

I only want to invite you to consider the amount and quality of the foods, you are already eating. The amount of food you eat, is determining how much energy you have to burn during the day. So, if you become more mindful of when you are no longer hungry, whilst eating, stop at this point, and you will already have reduced your food intake.

If you want to change more than just the amount of food, you eat, I encourage you to choose high quality food products. Your body is like a car, and if you fuel it with the right or a high-quality petrol, it will run better. Your engine certainly deserves the petrol-version of Power Plus! The quality of the meat and the vegetables, you buy has a great significance for the energy level you have during the day. This is also relevant for the cake and the chocolate, you eat! Three small bites of a high-quality chocolate is enjoyment to your body. Your body does not have to eat the WHOLE Toblerone but will enjoy just a few pieces.

Do you fuel your body with high-quality foods?

Recommended for optimal health is to consider the answer to the question "is what I am about to put into my mouth doing my body good or bad?" every time you are about to eat something. And if the answer is "bad", consider keeping your mouth closed.

My 5th piece of advice: ENJOYMENT and LOVE

My final piece of advice is also very important, because human beings have a basic need to seek pleasure, and we are deeply dependent on social connection to survive.

Newborn babies will die without physical contact, eye contact and care, and there is a reason that we are chasing likes on social media; human beings are not living well without nurturing, and our placement in the top of the food chain is due to our ability to collaborate with each other, and to cultivate each other, especially our love relationships.

Enjoyment and care come in many disguises, and we are often participating in social gatherings with an abundance of food and sweets.

"The Enjoyment Barometer"

A pitfall with enjoyment is, that we often tend to forget to push the STOP button, once we have pushed START. If we have opened the package of Toblerone, we tend to eat the whole thing, not attending to the level of enjoyment we feel, as we eat it.

Use an Enjoyment Barometer such as the one below and mark every bite you take from the Toblerone. Life is boring without the Toblerone, but if your enjoyment level is lower than 7, the calories are not worth taking in. The Enjoyment Barometer can be used with ALL your intakes of foods, and drinks and sweets. You can even use the barometer in all your personal relations, and in our daily activities.

The Enjoyment Barometer numbers from 1 to 10

1	2	3	4	5	6	7	8	9	10

How often are you enjoying what you take in, and what you observe around you?

Recommended for optimal health is to surround yourself with the people you care the most about and pay attention to feel enjoyment every day – both in your relationships and in the sweets, you choose to intake.

Onward Journey

Now you have been through "the theory". If this book was the theoretical basis of getting a driver's license, your ability to drive a car would be worth little before the practice got going.

To make it work, you must get to work.

If you have not yet started Level 1, today is a really good time. If you have been on it for a while, or have tried it in the past, you are already experienced, and now is a good time to build on those experiences.

I have more than 40 years of experience with running and training. When I was 12 to the age of 28, I had a personal trainer I met several times a week, I had a group I trained with in a club, that helped me on a day-to-day level. I have been fortunate to represent the Danish National Team 17 times, and the commitment to my trainer, my training partners, my club, and my country, was the daily support and motivation, especially on the days where training was hard to get done.

Today I also need an accountability partner to get my training done.

Despite all the years of experience, that I have, I sense a big difference to how much training I get done whether I have an accountability partner or not. I am in no way ashamed of this, and you should not be either.

If your training did not work up until now, I bet it is because you do not have an accountability partner.

Couch Potato Fitness (Online) Movement

There are several resources ready to support you in your upcoming lifestyle change. The digital resources are a helping hand to the work you have to do with yourself together with an accountability partner.

On the website www.couchpotatofitness.org there are resources available, to support your training. And those resources are very useful for you!

The community also has a Facebook-group, you can find via the website where you should add yourself to find news and inspiration.

The Facebook-group is the perfect place to find yourself an accountability partner, you can post your experiences, and ask questions for support. Here you can also keep yourself up to date on all initiatives regarding Couch Potato Fitness.

If you are more to using Instagram, you can find inspiration at @onekayaday.

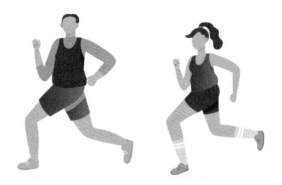

You have now learned a training program that you can use for the rest of your life. Even though the training focus is on physical exercise, I am sure that you have discovered how it is a question of exercising your psychology. If you have followed the program, you will have felt changes on your body firsthand, and how the physical exercises change your psychology because of the design of the program.

The key take home message of this book is that persistence is key. And the way to be persistent is … well, being persistent. All the artful and cunning plans you can make to catch yourself NOT getting into the traps of excuses and being lazy are allowed! Because the question is not IF you experience setbacks in and periods without training, but WHEN they will happen, and for HOW LONG they will happen to you.

Life hits us all in the head.

Illness. Injury. Busy times. Family increase. Whatever it may be, the art is to know the plan to GET BACK INTO the habit of training when you have left it momentarily.

And here is when your psychology plays the largest role.

> ➢ Are you telling yourself that you failed, and not – for God knows which time! – have played truant because you are lazy?

> Or are you telling yourself that you just have to start again, because breaks in training is a natural part of being human?

The more times you have practiced starting over with your training, the better you become at it. And the more training you do, the longer the time between your setbacks will be.

Success is ONLY a matter of starting over again.

It is simple but not easy. Use this book and start again from page 1. For the 20th time.

There is absolutely NO reason to be ashamed of breaks in your training if you start again as soon as possible.

Every new Day 1 is one day closer to a complete 30-day challenge, and that is a solid step. I hope that you have learned a lot about yourself, your psychology and your innate preferences about your training and your health. Changing your behavior is THE hardest thing human beings can do, and I hope that you have experienced more joys and successes than downturns the past 15 weeks. Irrespective of your experiences, you are now a stronger and healthier version of you if you have been through one or more of the three levels.

You can be proud of yourself for doing something about your health and prolonging your life

I hope that you will go through the material as many times as you need. You are invited to turn to Couch Potato Fitness every time it is needed, and use the principles as many times, as needed. Small steps is a key to success.

Repetitions will only make you more experienced and add steps to your health benefits. Regardless of your experiences, I would love to hear about them! One of the biggest joys of my work is when I hear about the changes, my athletes experience.

As a finishing remark, let me express my biggest appreciation to you, dear reader, because you have trusted me to read this far.

With the warmest and sincerest regards from Christina

Can You Help?

Thank You For Reading My Book!

I really appreciate all of your feedback, and I would LOVE hearing what you have to say about it. I always strive to improve, and I need your input to make the next version of this book and my future books better.

So I invite you please to leave me a review on Amazon letting me know what you thought of the book. A positive review makes me happy, and criticism will improve the next version – so that also makes me happy.

Thanks so much!

Christina Schnohr

Can I Help You?

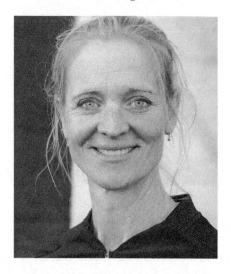

So I also want to make sure that you are not left wanting more! So if you are dedicated and ready to invest more, I also coach athletes 1:1.

Click here to access my calendar for a ½ hour call.

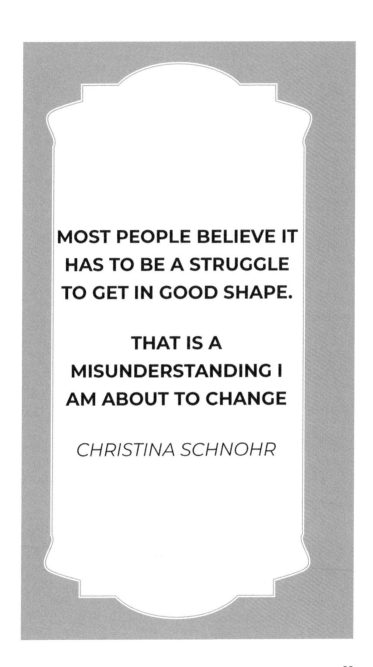

MOST PEOPLE BELIEVE IT
HAS TO BE A STRUGGLE
TO GET IN GOOD SHAPE.

THAT IS A
MISUNDERSTANDING I
AM ABOUT TO CHANGE

CHRISTINA SCHNOHR

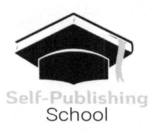

NOW IT'S YOUR TURN

Discover the EXACT 3-step blueprint you need to become a bestselling author in as little as 3 months.

Self-Publishing School helped me, and now
I want them to help you with this FREE
resource to begin outlining your book**!**

Even if you're busy, bad at writing, or don't know where to start, you CAN write a bestseller and build your best life.

With tools and experience across a variety of niches and professions, Self-Publishing School is the <u>only</u> resource you need to take your book to the finish line!

DON'T WAIT

Say "YES" to becoming a bestseller:

https://self-publishingschool.com/friend/

Follow the steps on the page to get a FREE resource to get started on your book and unlock a discount to get started with Self-Publishing School

Printed in Great Britain
by Amazon